# THE NO DIETING APPROACH; The best way to lose sufficient weight without dieting.

By John Reynold

Table of content

# Chapter 1

## Developing a success mindset to achieve your goals

What do you believe it takes to reach your goals? Hard work? Lots of actions? While both are crucial to become successful in accomplishing our objectives, none of them are attainable without a positive mentality.

As humans, we naturally tend to lean towards a pessimistic view when it comes to our goals and ambitions. We are prone to thinking that we have constraints either from inside ourselves or from other circumstances limiting us from genuinely reaching to where we want to be in life.

Our inclination to assume that we'll "believe it when we see it" shows that our attitudes are centered on our objectives not actually being feasible until they've been attained. The issue with this is that this typical thinking supports our limiting ideas and demonstrates a lack of trust in ourselves.

***The Success Mindset***

Success in reaching our objectives boils down to a 'success mindset'. Successful mindsets are ones focused on triumph, based on positive mental attitudes, powerful impulses and excellent habits. Acquiring a success attitude is the sure-fire technique to greatly boost your probability to accomplish your objectives.

The concept that attaining our objectives comes down to our habits and activities is really a normal sort of thinking that ignores a fundamental point; that our attitude is, in reality, the determiner of our energy and what actions we do. A negative thinking will tend to induce bad behaviors and similarly if we have a mindset that will only set into action once we have 'proof' that our objectives are possible, then the journey will be much longer and difficult. This is why, instead of thinking "I'll believe it when I see it", a success mentality will think "I'll see it when I believe it."

### *The Placebo Effect and What It Shows Us About The Power of Mindset*

The placebo effect is a fantastic illustration of how thought truly can be powerful. In scientific experiments, a set of volunteers were informed they got medicine that would treat a disease but were really given a sugar tablet that accomplishes nothing (the placebo) (the placebo). Yet after the study the participants claimed it's had a favorable impact - occasionally even healed their disease even if nothing has altered. This is the power of attitude.

How can we apply this to our goals? Well, when we create goals and ambitions how often do we actually think they'll come to fruition? Have 100% trust that they can be achieved? Have a totally unshakeable expectation?

Most of us don't because we hang on to negative thoughts and limiting ideas about ourselves that prohibit us from completely thinking we are competent or that it's at all conceivable. We prefer to listen to the ideas of others despite them misaligning with our own or bend to social influences that make us feel we should think and behave a specific way.

There are various reasons why we hold different sorts of mindsets yet a success attitude may be developed.

### ***How to develop a success mindset***

People with a success mindset have a unique way of viewing things. They have optimistic outlooks and are able to put trust totally in their abilities to achieve. With that in mind, here are a few techniques that may change a negative mentality into a successful one.

*1. A Success Mindset Comes From a Growth Mindset*

How does a mentality even present itself? It arises from the way you speak to yourself in the solitude of your own brain. Realising this will go a long way towards recognizing how you communicate to yourself and people around you. If it's mostly negative language you use when you speak about your objectives and desires then this is an example of a stuck mentality.

A negative mindset carries with it a great amount of limiting beliefs. It produces a stuck mentality — one that can't look beyond its own constraints. A growth mentality perceives these constraints and seeks beyond them - it discovers solutions to overcome barriers and thinks that this will result in success.

When you think about your objective, a fixed mentality may consider "what if I fail? " A development mentality would look at the same aim and say "failures happen but that doesn't imply I won't be successful."

There's a lot of power in shifting your viewpoint.

2. *Look For The Successes*

It's incredibly crucial to get your thoughts focused on positive parts of your aim. Finding inspiration via others may be incredibly motivating and keep you on track with establishing your success mentality; reaffirming your confidence that your ambitions can be attained. Find individuals who you can discuss with about how they attained their objectives and seek out and surround yourself with positive people. This is vital if you're learning to create a positive mentality.

3. *Eliminate Negativity*

You might come up against a lot of negativity occasionally either from other people or inside yourself. Understanding that other people's negative perceptions are produced via their own fears and limiting beliefs can go a long way in keeping your success mentality. But for a lot of us, negative talk may arise from inside and they generally materialize as negative phrases such as can't, won't, shouldn't. Sometimes, when we think about how we're going to attain our objectives, words in our brains come out as negative absolutes: 'It never works out for me' or 'I always fail.'

When you detect these coming up you need to flip them around with 'It always works out for me!

' and 'I never fail!

’ The secret is to trust it no matter what’s occurred in the past. Remember that every new day is a clean slate and for you to modify your mentality.

*4. Create a Vision*

Envisioning your final objective and seeing it in your head is a crucial quality of a success mentality. Allowing oneself to picture our triumph provides a great enthusiasm that shouldn’t be underestimated. When our brain gets thrilled at the notion of accomplishing our objectives, we become more devoted, work more towards achieving it and more inclined to do whatever it takes to make it happen.

If this entails constructing a vision board that you can glance at to remind yourself every day then go for it. Small strategies like these go a long way in preserving your success mentality and shouldn't be overlooked.

*5. Build your experience by learning from your errors and failures*

learn from loss

One of the greatest methods to establish a success mentality is via developing your experiences by learning from your errors and disappointments.

First, you have to accept errors and failures as feedback. Sadly, most people don't look at them this way.

Most individuals are so terrified to make errors that they don't even dare to attempt.

They realize that if they want to attain financial independence, they need to learn to start a company or learn to invest.

However, most of them don't take any action on this because they let their fear of failure stop them.

From now on, look at errors and failures as experiences. The more experience you get, the better you become.

Like when you are playing games, the more monsters and opponents you battle, the more experience you acquire and consequently, the higher your level rises.

Therefore, don't be scared to make errors or to fail.

And remember, failure is not the reverse of success, it is part of achievement.

*6. Put yourself in a new demanding and unpleasant circumstance*

challenge yourself, If you truly want to build yourself and create a better attitude for success, you must push yourself to do the tough from time to time.

Most individuals are terrified of change. They like to remain in their comfort zone, and they don't dare to step out of it.

Staying in your comfort zone and doing what you have always done is wonderful, but it will never yield you the spectacular outcomes you seek.

Thus, from time to time, push yourself to do something unpleasant.

Put yourself in a stressful scenario so that you will teach your mind to think and behave differently.

After all, what doesn't kill you makes you stronger.

Read the autobiographies of successful individuals and you will discover that amazing people are able to attain great outcomes in life because they have gone through significant disappointments and tribulations.

It is the path that forms their personalities.

Without the voyage, they would never become who they are.

And the same applies to you. If you continue to remain inside your comfort zone, you will never progress to a higher level.

*7. Keep a success notebook and examine your victories from time to time*

individuals who succeed have momentum
One fantastic technique to cultivate a success attitude is to continually remind yourself that you are a winner.

You want to program nice and optimistic ideas to your mind to retain your confidence.

And you may do so by maintaining a success diary so that you can examine your achievements from time to time.

As human beings, we are continually touched by our emotions.

Whenever you are sad, glance at your success notebook and remind yourself of all the excellent things you have done.

It doesn't matter how large or tiny your successes are. The idea is to consistently train your mind with optimistic thoughts.

You want to remind yourself that you are a champion and that you can accomplish it no matter how bad the conditions get.

It is like what Tony Robbins said:

"People who succeed have momentum. The more they succeed, the more they want to succeed, and the more they find a way to achieve. Similarly, when someone is sinking, the inclination is to embark on a downward cycle that may even become a self-fulfilling prophecy."

So, you want to place yourself on the upward spiral by keeping your momentum.

This is why you want to keep a record of your wins and victories. Every time when you question yourself or when you feel low, glance at your success diary.

Let your previous triumphs enhance your future successes.

*8. Surround yourself with the greatest people.*
One of the most effective techniques to swiftly build up your success attitude is to surround yourself with the finest.

When you communicate and have discussions with people, you will be impacted by their thinking and opinions.

That said, if you surround yourself with substandard people, you will think like they do.

For instance, you will play the blame game, pointing fingers, and offer awful excuses every time you make a mistake or fail.

On the contrary, when you surround yourself with successful people, guess what you will be talking about?

If you join a group of businessmen, you will discuss business and economics.

You will never speak about who's being fired or what your boss did to make you despise him.

Instead, you will debate and chat about business.

This is how surrounding yourself with high talent can influence the way you think.

So, start creating new acquaintances and spend more time establishing ties with other successful individuals.

It is crucial to surround oneself with the people who you look up to and who you aspire to be in the future..

### *9. Take your enthusiasm and expertise and play it to the next level*

Adore what you do If you want to level up and increase your outcomes, you must learn to dive deep with your enthusiasm.

You have to raise your abilities to the next level by playing all out to produce something outstanding.Don’t merely enjoy what you do, elevate it to a greater level.

For example, if you are an author, what can you do to move your work to the next level?

Perhaps, if you are producing articles at 1,000 words on average, then you may want to try publishing an ultimate guide of 5,000 or even more words.The objective is to make it huge and take your enthusiasm to a greater level.

So, you are enthusiastic about baking? Then maybe you can make something unique and unusual like when you split the cake into halves, you receive a duplicate of a Facebook logo within the cake.

Doing the same thing will just bring you the same old outcome.If you wish to acquire anything different, you will have to play the game differently.Most individuals are not successful because they are doing regular things that most people do.Amazing individuals, on the other hand, do something extra so that they may become extraordinary.

Ask yourself, what can you do to elevate your passion to a greater level? How do you do something unusual and play it big?

### *10. Define your standards and accept nothing less*

Developing a success mentality has a lot to say about your degree of acceptance.
There is no way you can become successful if you don't boost your expectations. Think about it, if you are someone who doesn't care about the quality of your material, yet you aim to establish an authoritative site, how can that be achievable, right?

It is like you want to be a champion, but you refuse to practice, and you are satisfied with substandard results. Successful individuals have their own standards. They know what type of outcomes they can tolerate and what they can't. And they will keep to their ideals and values.

Whenever they provide sub-par work, they will work on their crafts again to better the quality.

Hence, identify your criteria, what you can tolerate, and what you can't.

Stick to your own ideals and never accept anything less than the level you have established. This is how you strive for excellence and deliver great results.

*11. Set intriguing objectives and work on them attentively*

One of the simplest methods to establish a success attitude in you is to pick an exciting goal that you look forward to and work on it carefully.

You don't need to have a lot of objectives, you just need to start with one. Identify a goal that you genuinely want to attain within 90 days, establish a strategy, and then work on it persistently. If you can fulfill this objective in 3 months, you are indirectly establishing the character you need for a larger success.

A lot of people don't establish objectives. Even if they do, they don't stick to their strategy. My idea is to start with something smaller. If you think you don't have the discipline or you feel it will never work because you constantly procrastinate, start small.

Maybe you can come up with a one-month objective. The idea is to give oneself a clear aim and direction to pursue. You want to teach your mind to live an intentional life. So that in the future, you may plan for higher success and attain better successes in life.

## *12. Trust your gut sense and heed to your inclination*

Listening to your gut instinct is an element of creating a success attitude.

You must learn to trust your gut because when you do, you may make better and more accurate judgments. According to this article from Harvard Business Review, gut sensations are signals from the insula and the amygdala in your brain. And those signals are feelings that something "feels" correct or bad.

Learning how to trust your gut emotions and instincts may be a significant aspect in your success in life. Now, I'm not saying analytical data is not vital, but you need to operate from both. You may do all the analyzes with your analytic mind, but you must also consider your feelings and emotions.

The more you teach yourself to listen to your instincts, the more self-aware you will become. And this helps you make better judgments in all you do.

*13. Keep making progress and avoid stagnation*

Development adds up to tremendous outcomes
Another strategy to establish a success attitude is to make sure you are continually making progress and not being stagnated. Regardless of whether you are making errors or going ahead, you must make progress each day.

If you remain static, you will rapidly lose your momentum and ultimately, buy into life in the comfort zone that you're in.

In order to continue to develop and progress, avoid stagnation. This will help you tackle new problems and increase your capacity to overcome barriers. You have learnt that you should push yourself from time to time. You realize that if you want to level up, you must play it full out and commit to doing something differently.

Plus, you also know that you may start with minor objectives and work on them steadily until you reach them. These are the progress you should be looking forward to accomplishing. Always have these great thoughts in your mind from Robin Sharma:

"Success is built via the execution of a few minor daily disciplines that build up over time to yield results well beyond what you could have ever planned for."

## *Conclusion*

Now that you understand what you can do to establish a success mentality. What you need to do next is to incorporate these 13 ways into your everyday life.

And please realize that creating a successful attitude might take time.

Hence, if you don't observe any substantial effect, don't lose hope. Trust yourself and go forth.

# Chapter 2

## Why lose weight?

The advantages of maintaining a healthy weight go well beyond greater energy and lower clothing sizes. By decreasing weight or maintaining a healthy weight, you are also likely to experience a superior quality-of-life too.

If you battle with your weight, you may very well know that the dressing room is one of the few locations that give you a brutal reality check. But is squeezing into a pair of jeans, swimwear, or even a good shirt one of the sole reasons to lose weight?

While, certainly, your weight may impact how you feel about yourself and even how others regard you, body image is not the only reason you should go on a weight-loss journey. In truth, for individuals who are overweight or obese, decreasing weight truly brings many advantages beyond looking fantastic in your new clothing.

Ultimately, being overweight has several negative effects, from simple things like back discomfort to more major implications like being more likely to develop type 2 diabetes.

Besides decreasing these health risks, there are also lots of little-known advantages that come with a trimmer body. Read on to learn some insights into how your body and lifestyle might alter after dropping some pounds.

You'll have all the more incentive to fight the bulge since experts have shown that when you come up with strong motives to lose weight before commencing on your trip, you lose more weight than those who are less driven!

### *1. You'll Have Less Joint Pain*

You know what we're talking about. Being overweight may put some considerable pressure on your joints—especially your knees. While everyone needs to cope with regular wear and tear on their joints, people who are overweight put up unnecessary stress on these same joints. On top of that, inflammatory elements that are related to weight increase might lead to problems in smaller joints, such as your hands. That's why an anti-inflammatory diet has been demonstrated to help relieve arthritic symptoms.

### *2. Get Offered Your Dream Job*

As immoral as it may sound, research has discovered that weight may even severely affect your chances of landing a job. In a study published in the International Journal of Obesity, researchers discovered that employment choices were influenced adversely when the picture showed a person who was overweight compared to a photo of the same person following weight-loss surgery.

Another analysis in Occupational Medicine & Health Affairs found that persons with high BMIs are commonly disregarded for initial job offers, supervisory roles, and promotions compared to their slimmer peers. Slimming down won't simply improve your interviewer's or boss' prejudice, it will also make you more confident—and make interviews a lot simpler!

### *3. Food Will Taste Better*

This is something you probably haven't heard before: After dumping your spare tire, your meal may taste even better. Researchers from Stanford University discovered that overweight persons had less taste sensitivity than their smaller counterparts, probably because their taste receptors grow blunted with misuse. Another idea speculates that hormonal modifications that take place with weight reduction may modify the way taste receptors interact with the brain.

### *4. You May Say 'Goodbye!' To Seasonal Allergy Suffering*

Do the first indications of Spring come with the dread of knowing you'll have to get out the eye drops and Kleenex? Turns out, your weight may be to blame for some of your symptoms. That's because being overweight puts a load on the adrenal glands and respiratory system, which may increase asthma and allergy symptoms. Trimming down might mean you'll finally be able to stroll outdoors and smell the flowers!

### *5. You'll Experience Fewer Colds*

Successful weight reduction generally comes with a lifestyle overhaul—one that involves getting a good night's rest, filling up with a micronutrient-dense diet heavy in fresh vegetables and whole grains, and working up a sweat frequently. According to Harvard Medical School, each of these modifications may assist to boost your immune system.

## *6. You Won't Sweat As Much*

Does it ever feel like you're in a sauna when it's only 70 degrees? It's because fat insulates the body and elevates core temperature, making you feel warmer than smaller people. For the same reason, overweight folks tend to sweat more. Drop the muffin top and you won't have to go directly to the bathroom to dry off after walking anywhere.

## *7. Your Complexion Will Clear Up*

Toss off those creams and serums! If you suffer from skin concerns such as psoriasis, eczema, or acne, reducing a few pounds may help your complexion clean up. That's because minerals present in nutritious diets have been demonstrated to offer beautifying qualities.

Not to mention, you're also probably shunning sugar, which is known to break down the amino acids in the proteins that keep skin appearing elastic and young: collagen and elastin.
Plus, if you're consuming more fiber and probiotics, such as yogurt with live active cultures, you're likely increasing your gut health as well.

Because our microbiome helps control our immune system, its health plays a crucial role in fighting inflammatory skin problems. Experts think that providing probiotics may assist to lower patients' levels of inflammatory proteins and improve skin disease symptoms.

### *8. You'll Gain Confidence*

That sensation you receive once you walk on the scale and realize you're 5 pounds lighter isn't simply relief. It's also the confidence in your success and in knowing you've taken charge of your life for the better—and you've got the results to show it.

One Reddit member, who shed 140 pounds came to the revelation that he wasn't an innately lazy person: "I've been overweight for much of my life and it always seemed like a moral failing. [...] I now know that being big makes you lazy. It aches to move, to stand, to live—no surprise all I wanted to do was lay down or sleep!" He says, "Being lazy didn't make me obese—I was lazy because I was fat."

### *9. People Will Be Nicer To You*

If it were up to us, it wouldn't be like this. But, the fact is, our culture frequently discriminates against overweight individuals, whether that means they'll attract less attention from healthcare professionals or receive more harsh remarks from peers. (It's scientifically proven!) But, when you've dropped weight, you'll start to notice things shift.

People who earlier disregarded you may welcome you with a grin or even offer to hold the door for you. "I have dropped 120 pounds already, and people treat me so much differently," comments a FatSecret message board member, another user agrees: "Sad, but true... it seems everyone is kinder to you [when you lose weight.]"

### *10. You'll Feel Energized*

After decreasing the pounds, you may immediately discover that you have considerably more energy. It's not only because you're consuming more items that sustain your energy levels. It's also because when you're dragging around less weight, your body requires less energy to keep you alive.

### *11. Your General Mood Will Improve*

It may be uncomfortable at first, but after you start dropping the pounds, exercising will become easier and less of a drain on your body. As a consequence, you'll receive one of its key advantages besides calorie burn: endorphins!

These feel-good chemicals that rush your body after a terrific spin class can substantially enhance your mood and get you hooked on those sweat sessions. Get the most out of pumping iron by fuelling yourself correctly.

### *12. You'll Try New Activities*

With all that excess weight, you may have been restricted in what sorts of workouts, hobbies, or even holidays you could go on. With a trimmer frame, look forward to indulging in outdoor sports you were never able to partake in previously like hiking, kayaking, skiing, mountain biking, surfing, or rock climbing. You can even get the entire family involved!

### *13. Your Cancer Risk Will Decrease*

Most people know that smoking and sunbathing may boost your cancer risk, but few people understand that obesity is associated with cancer, too. (Experts think that the same inflammation that promotes weight gain causes DNA damage and the consequent illnesses.) That's terrible news.

The good news, however, is that you may lower levels of inflammation by decreasing only five percent of your body weight, according to a Cancer Research study of postmenopausal women.

### *14. You'll Live Longer*

You may have already guessed, but a slimmer you correlates to a lower chance of sickness, and therefore, a longer life. We know you don't need much evidence, but you may not have to know the degree fat causes an influence on your longevity; A meta-analysis of 20 research, published in PLOS Medicine, found that excessive obesity may lower your life expectancy by up to 14 years!

Those who are overweight or obese who lose 3 percent of their weight may not only notice health advantages but may also prolong their life by two years, according to the British National Institute for Health and Care Excellence.

### *15. Your sexual desire would grow*

Leave the bedroom blues behind. As your BMI falls, you'll more easily become aroused. It's all attributable to the surge in testosterone levels that comes with torching away body fat.

In a study published in the Journal of Clinical Endocrinology & Metabolism, heavier men had T-levels comparable to elderly gents nearly a full decade older. Other research has revealed that women with belly fat buildup had higher levels of cortisol, a stress hormone.

More cortisol—and consequently greater stress levels—was shown to interfere with sexual desire. Besides what's going on with your body on the inside, lowering that muffin top may help you to feel less self-conscious in the nude, which might improve your urge to get it on as well.

### *16. And You'll Enjoy It More!*

A Duke University Medical Center assessment of 1,210 persons of varied weights revealed that obese people were 25 times more likely to indicate unhappiness with their time between the sheets than their thinner counterparts. The good news? Shedding a little 10 percent decrease in your body weight was found to boost sexual pleasure. So you might even enjoy the perks in the bedroom before you've attained your ideal weight!

# Chapter 3

## Reason most people are sick and overweight and how to avoid it

Obesity is one of the largest health issues in the globe.
It's connected with other related disorders, generally known as metabolic syndrome. These include increased blood pressure, raised blood sugar and a bad blood lipid profile.

People with metabolic syndrome are at a considerably increased risk of heart disease and type 2 diabetes, compared to those whose weight is in a normal range.
Over the last decades, considerable study has focused on the causes of

obesity and how it may be avoided or treated.

### *Obesity and Willpower*

Many individuals appear to assume that weight gain and obesity are caused by a lack of willpower.
That's not fully accurate. Although weight growth is mostly a product of eating behavior and lifestyle, certain individuals are at a disadvantage when it comes to managing their eating habits.
The truth is, overeating is influenced by different biological variables including heredity and hormones. Certain folks are just inclined to accumulate weight.

Of course, individuals may overcome their inherited disadvantages by modifying their lifestyle and behavior. Lifestyle changes need effort, focus and patience. Nevertheless, statements that conduct is entirely a result of willpower is much too simple. They don't take into consideration all the other elements that ultimately decide what individuals do and when they do it.

Here are 10 variables that are primary drivers of weight gain, obesity and metabolic illness, many of which have little to do with willpower.

1. *Genetics*
Obesity has a substantial hereditary component. Children of parents with obesity are far more likely to have obesity than children of lean parents. That doesn't imply that obesity is fully predestined. What you consume may have a huge influence on which genes are expressed and which are not.

Non-industrialized civilizations quickly gain obese when they start eating a standard Western diet. Their DNA didn't change, but the environment and the signals they transmitted to their genes changed. Put simply, genetic components do impact your propensity to acquiring weight. Studies on identical twins reveal this extremely clearly.

Summary; Some persons seem to be genetically sensitive to weight gain and obesity.

*2. Engineered Junk Foods*

Heavily processed meals are typically nothing more than refined components coupled with additives. These items are meant to be inexpensive, stay long on the market and taste so fantastically delicious that they are hard to refuse.

By making meals as appetizing as possible, food makers are striving to enhance sales. But they also promote overeating. Most processed foods nowadays don't resemble real foods at all. These are carefully developed items, meant to get consumers hooked.

Summary; Stores are packed with packaged foods that are hard to resist. These products also increase overeating.

*3. Food Addiction*

Many sugar-sweetened, high-fat junk meals trigger the reward centers in your brain.

In fact, these meals are frequently linked to widely misused narcotics including alcohol, cocaine, nicotine and cannabis.

Junk foods may induce addiction in vulnerable people. These individuals lose control over their eating habit, comparable to persons battling with alcohol addiction losing control over their drinking activity.

Addiction is a complicated condition that may be extremely tough to overcome. When you get addicted to anything, you lose your freedom of choice and the biochemistry in your brain begins calling the shots for you.

Summary;
Some individuals have extreme eating cravings or addiction. This notably applies to sugar-sweetened, high-fat junk meals which trigger the reward centers in the brain.

## *4. Aggressive Marketing*

Junk food makers are incredibly active marketers.
Their practices might turn dishonest at times and they occasionally attempt to advertise highly harmful items as healthy meals.
These firms also make deceptive promises. What's worse, they direct their advertisements exclusively at youngsters.
In today's environment, children are growing obese and getting diabetic and hooked to junk foods long before they're mature enough to make educated judgments about these things.

Summary; Food companies spend a lot of money promoting bad food, sometimes explicitly targeting youngsters, who don't have the knowledge and experience to recognize they are being deceived.

### *5. Insulin*

Insulin is a highly essential hormone that controls energy storage, among other things.

One of its roles is to signal fat cells to store fat and to hang on to the fat they currently contain.

The Western diet induces insulin resistance in many overweight and those with obesity. This boosts insulin levels all across the body, causing energy to be stored in fat cells instead of being accessible for utilization.

While insulin's function in obesity is debatable, some studies imply that elevated insulin levels have a causal impact in the development of obesity.

One of the greatest strategies to reduce your insulin is to cut down on simple or refined carbs while boosting fiber consumption. This generally leads to a spontaneous decrease in calorie intake and uncomplicated weight loss – no calorie tracking or portion management required.

Summary; High insulin levels and insulin resistance are connected to the development of obesity. To decrease insulin levels, cut your consumption of refined carbohydrates and consume more fiber.

*6. Certain Medications*

Many pharmacological medicines might induce weight gain as a side effect.

For example, antidepressants have been related to mild weight increase over time.

Other examples are diabetic medicine and antipsychotics.

These medications don't reduce your willpower. They influence the operation of your body and brain,

decreasing metabolic rate or raising hunger.
Summary Some drugs may cause weight gain by lowering the quantity of calories expended or boosting hunger.

*7. Leptin Resistance*
Leptin is another hormone that plays a significant function in obesity.
It is generated by fat cells and its blood levels rise with increased fat mass. For this reason, leptin levels are notably high in patients with obesity.
In healthy persons, increased leptin levels are connected to decreased appetite. When performing correctly, it should signal your brain how high your fat reserves are.

The trouble is that leptin isn't operating as it should in many individuals who have obesity, since for some reason it cannot penetrate the

blood-brain barrier. This syndrome is termed leptin resistance and is thought to be a key role in the pathophysiology of obesity.
Summary Leptin, an appetite-reducing hormone, doesn't function in many persons who have obesity.

*8. Food Availability*

Another element that greatly increases people's waistline is food availability, which has expanded tremendously in the previous several centuries.
Food, particularly junk food, is omnipresent today. Shops showcase appealing meals where they are most likely to attract your attention.
Another difficulty is that junk food is typically cheaper than nutritious, whole meals, particularly in America.

Some individuals, particularly in impoverished districts, don't even have the choice of buying actual goods, such as fresh fruit and vegetables.
Convenience shops in these locations exclusively offer drinks, candies and processed, packaged junk meals.
How can it be a question of choice if there is none?

Summary;
In certain locations, acquiring fresh, healthful meals may be difficult or costly, giving consumers little alternative except to purchase harmful junk foods.

*9. Sugar*
Added sugar may be the single worst component of the contemporary diet.
That's because sugar alters the hormones and biochemistry of your

body when taken in excess. This, in turn, adds to weight growth.
Added sugar is half glucose, half fructose. People receive glucose from a number of meals, including carbohydrates, but the bulk of fructose comes from added sugar.

Excess fructose consumption may promote insulin resistance and increased insulin levels. It also doesn't produce satiety in the same way glucose does.
For all these reasons, sugar leads to increased energy storage and, eventually, obesity.
Summary Scientists think that high sugar consumption may be one of the primary reasons for obesity.

*10. Misinformation*
People all across the globe are being deceived about health and nutrition.

There are various causes behind this, but the issue mostly hinges on where individuals acquire their information from.

Many books, for example, promote incomplete or even false information regarding health and diet.
Some news sources also oversimplify or misrepresent the outcomes of scientific research and the results are usually presented out of context.

Other information may simply be old or based on assumptions that have never been completely confirmed.
Food corporations also have a role.
Some market things, such as weight reduction pills, that do not work.

Weight loss tactics based on erroneous information might hold back your progress. It's crucial to pick your sources properly.

Summary Misinformation may lead to weight gain in certain persons. It may also make weight reduction more challenging.

### *The Bottom Line*

If you have worries about your waistline, you should not take this article as an excuse to quit.

While you can't totally control the way your body operates, you can learn how to regulate your eating habits and adjust your lifestyle.
Unless there is any medical ailment coming in your way, it is within your capacity to regulate your weight.
It sometimes requires hard effort and a major lifestyle adjustment, but many individuals do succeed in the long

term despite having the odds stacked against them.

The objective of this book is to open people's eyes to the reality that something other than individual responsibility plays a part in the obesity pandemic.
The reality is that current eating habits and food culture must be adjusted to be able to reverse this situation on a worldwide basis.

The concept that it is all caused by a lack of willpower is precisely what food manufacturers want you to think, so they can continue their marketing in peace.

# Chapter 4

## Secrets and tips to a successful weight loss

Here are some secrets and recommendations that can assist you to manage your weight-reduction plan. These are nuggets of information, methods, tips, and recommendations that we've found useful while attempting to reduce or maintain weight and build a better routine of eating.

- Take tiny steps.

You need nice hiking boots and stronger legs to climb a mountain. You don't climb a mountain without preparedness. You'll want to break down your large goal of weight reduction into mini-goals that carry you to the top, like sleeping 7-8 hours a night or cutting out your nocturnal munching at 8 p.m. To set yourself up for success, before you even write down your objectives, step one should be acquiring tools, such as a scale, meal prep containers, or a blender for producing weight-loss smoothies.

- Have a plan.

While having a daily or weekly plan can help you lay out your days so you can reach your goals, you can start with something as easy as reading up on the 7 Must-Buy Foods on a Healthy Grocery List, According to a Dietitian before you go shopping to ensure that you have every ingredient you need to improve health and lose weight.

- Drink additional water and tea.

Drinking smoothies as meal replacements don't fulfill your daily fluid needs. We'd want to see you drink roughly 64 ounces of water each day. Remember, part of the water may come from meals, especially vegetables and fruits.

Tea and coffee contribute but beware of the calorie impact you might take if you add lumps of sugar or tablespoons of creamer.

Brewed green, white, or black teas are rich with substances called catechins, belly-fat crusaders that blast belly fat by revving the metabolism, boosting the release of fat from fat cells, and speeding up the liver's fat-burning ability.

- Don't starve yourself.

Skipping meals tends to backfire on you. You feel so hungry that you lose all control and devour the nearest, most calorie-dense meal you can locate, eat too quickly, and overeat. Instead, be attentive to your hunger. Satisfy it with a smoothie or high-fiber food like cut-up veggies or a high-protein snack like a hard-boiled egg, cheese stick, or a handful of nuts and seeds.

- Push breakfast back.

Instead of gobbling down breakfast at home, eat at your desk a couple of hours later than you regularly do. Pushing out your first meal of the day automatically limits your "eating window"—the number of hours you spend each day snacking.

Why is that beneficial? Sticking to a narrower eating window may help you lose weight, even if you consume more food throughout the day, research published in the journal Cell Metabolism revealed.

Reaching this discovery, researchers placed groups of mice on a high-fat, high-calorie diet for 100 days. Half of them were permitted to nibble throughout the night and day on a healthy, restricted diet whereas the others only had access to food for eight hours, but could eat anything they wanted. Oddly enough, the fasting mice maintained thin whereas the mice that noshed around the clock got obese—even though both groups ingested the same amount of calories.

- Get a dog and hoof it.

Studies show that individuals who keep dogs are healthier and fitter than those who don't, since walking a dog is a decent forced regular activity. You'll burn 61 calories in only 15 minutes of walking a dog, according to the American College of Sports Medicine.

- Become a label reader.

One of the finest ways to practice mindful eating is to become a student of the nutrition information panel on packaged goods. By constantly reviewing the nutrition label (and don't forget the ingredients page!), you'll be more inclined to make better food choices. You'll be shocked at how frequently you will put a product back on the shop shelf after reading unpronounceable words on the ingredients list.

- Sprinkle on some vinegar.

Adding a few tablespoons of vinegar to a sandwich or salad might limit the body's absorption of carbs and diminish sensations of hunger so you eat less. Studies have indicated that vinegar consumed with a carb-heavy meal may minimize blood sugar rises by a fifth or more.

- Bag it.

Pack your lunch to take to work every day and you will avoid the temptation of calorie-dense fast-food restaurant selections. Research in the journal Journal of the American Academy of Nutrition and Dietetics indicated that 92% of meals from large-chain and local restaurants contain more calories than is advised for the typical individual.

Bringing a nutritious lunch to work might save you hundreds of calories every week. Also, try these 7 Healthy Lunch Habits For A Flat Belly.

- Go to sleep sooner to wake up early.

According to experts, late sleepers—defined as individuals who get up around 10:45 a.m.—consume 248 more calories throughout the day, as well as half as many fruits and vegetables and double the amount of fast food as those who set their alarm earlier. If these results seem disturbing to you night owls, consider setting your alarm clock 15 minutes earlier each day until you're getting out of bed at a more normal hour. This may take a week or so but it works.

- Walk, don't sit.

While your eating choices have a higher effect on weight growth or reduction than exercise will, don't overlook the significant advantages of moving more every day.

When you are physically active, your body metabolizes food more effectively, you grow muscle, you sleep better, and you feel happier. All of these might affect your weight reduction. So make sure to obtain at least 30 minutes of physical exercise a day. Start by using the stairs instead of the elevator.

According to a University of New Mexico Health Sciences Center research, a person who weighs 150 pounds might lose around six pounds per year merely by moving up two flights of stairs every day.

Chapter 5

## Fitness strategy; Weight loss exercises at home

Exercise is vital for your overall health. Good health and weight reduction are associated. If a person has a higher body mass index, then they are prone to many ailments including hypertension, diabetes, cholesterol, and other cardiovascular issues. Exercise becomes also extremely vital for the successful treatment of these disorders.

An essential component that needs to be addressed to reduce weight is exercise. In your normal routine, if you follow your diet and neglect exercise then you will find your body responding extremely differently.

Exercise has various advantages associated with it along with weight reduction. Exercise boosts your mood, strengthens your bones, and decreases the risk of numerous chronic illnesses. People prefer to pull themselves out from exercising as they won't have the time to go to the gym or perhaps cannot afford to join a gym or have personal trainers to lead them on their fitness path.

## Best Exercises to Lose Weight At Home

So, here we would like to offer you the greatest and most popular fitness programs that you may do at home and make yourself stronger, fitter, and healthier.

***1. Aerobic Exercises***

Walking is considered one of the best weight loss exercises. Walking at a fast pace is a great exercise for burning calories. An exercise program that puts minimal stress on your joints and can be incorporated into your day-to-day activities.

According to many studies, A 70-kg individual burns around 167 calories per 30 minutes of walking at a pace of 6.4 kph. It is also observed that an individual can reduce their body fat by an average of 1.5% and waist circumference by 2.8 cm by walking for 50-70 minutes 3 times per week.

Jogging and Running are considered to be the king of weight loss exercises. These exercises are total body-integrated exercises. It will strengthen your legs and be very effective for belly fat. The primary difference between running and jogging is the pace. Jogging is between 6 – 9 kph and running will be about 10 kph.

Running and Jogging will roughly help burn 372 calories per 30 minutes and 298 calories per 30 minutes respectively. The combination of these 3 workouts will undoubtedly assist enhance your muscle strength and general body weight to keep you fit and healthy.

## Exercise Pattern

Set aside 1 hour of your time and integrate these workouts into your program.

Start with walking exercises for 15 minutes.
Increase your pace and start Jogging for the following 15 minutes.
With a continual rise in speed, run for another 15 minutes.
Reduce your pace and come back to jogging for 10 minutes.
Relax your body and slow down your speed and walk for 5 minutes.

### *2. Skipping or Jumping Rope*

Skipping exercise delivers a whole-body workout and helps boost your muscular power, and metabolism, and burns many calories in a short period.

Skipping exercises done frequently would bring in tranquility and assist to reduce sadness and anxiety. The exercise also boosts your heart rate which leads to quicker pumping of blood throughout your body to maintain your heart in a healthier and healthy state. Along with your heart, physical activity takes care of your lungs by keeping them functional and healthy.

Everybody has a unique physique and this causes the method to produce varied outcomes. Losing weight is nothing but burning more calories than you ingest and skipping would undoubtedly help you achieve so. This sort of workout typically burns calories close to 1300 every hour.

Exercise Pattern

On a flat surface, stand with your back straight.
Make sure your feet are together and pointing straight.

Keep your hand straight pointing downwards near your thighs.
Jump off the ground and let your rope pass under your feet and bring it back.
Repeat these procedures and improve your leaping speed continually.

### *3. Planks*

Plank Pose or Plank exercise is one of the most effective full-body exercises. The primary benefit of Plank's exercise is it addresses most of the major muscle groups in the body. It strengthens your muscles in the core, shoulder, arms, chest, back, and hips. Along with these advantages, Plank workouts aid in swiftly burning the extra fats and calories from the body.

An exercise that looks to be a basic and easy one but it's strenuous and hard. The plank exercise is a perfect illustration of the longer you train the greater will be your outcomes. You need to concentrate on keeping your plank posture for a longer duration to get rapid and greater results.

Plank exercise includes many variants that target different muscles and body parts. Each variant is highly useful and maintains the development of your core strength, body balance, endurance, and posture.

Plank Exercise Variations;

The Standard Plank:
It is also known as The Extended Arms Plank. This posture is best suited for novices who are looking forward to strengthening their core strength. This exercise is fantastic for boosting metabolic activity and digestion. The forearm Plank variant is an identical form of the extended arms plank. The target areas of this

exercise are the core, arms, shoulders, and back.

The Mountain Climbers:

Considered one of the difficult variants of plank training. A full-body exercise that burns extra calories and fat from the body. The targeted regions of this exercise include the biceps, hamstring muscles, core, triceps, and chest.

*Exercise Pattern*

Get down into the Push-Up or Standard Plank Position.

Now bend your right knee and draw it towards your chest.

Push your right knee back to your original position.

Now bend your left knee and get it near your chest.

Push your left knee back to your original posture

Continue the aforementioned steps roughly 20-25 times.

The Reverse Plank:

This is a version of the conventional plank but done in a reverse way. This exercise is a wonderful method to extend your body. An exercise that removes unneeded fats and calories from your body. It aids in strengthening your core, shoulders, back, chest, and gluteal muscles.

*Exercise Pattern*

Sit down and stretch your legs in front of you.
Place your hands behind your hips for your upper body support.
Now elevate your hips by straightening your hand and making a straight line with your body.
Hold this posture for 40-60 seconds.

Repeat these processes and approaches roughly 20-30 times.

### *4. Push-Ups and Pull-Ups*

Push-ups are one of the most popular workouts and it is a workout that can be done at any time, anywhere, and by everyone. Push-up exercise is highly good for weight reduction since it pushes your body away from the ground and exerts energy which in turn burns calories.

Push-up workouts are helpful since it burns calories rapidly and puts you concentrate on the bigger muscles in your upper body. Push-up training also works on your chest, shoulders, back, biceps, and triceps. Push-up exercises can help develop your core muscles and make your body physically sturdy and healthy.

Push-ups aid in growing lean muscles in our chest, shoulders, biceps, and triceps. If you keep exercising push-ups for weeks or months or years, then you will grow a big quantity of muscle mass, and to retain your muscle your body needs to waste its calories.

*Exercise Pattern*

Look for anti-slippery and level surfaces.
Place your hands pointing ahead and slightly wider than your shoulder width.
Set your feet together or slightly apart in a comfortable posture. Initially, you may keep your feet apart until you discover a healthy balance.
Now lower your shoulders as low as possible towards the floor and push up back and straighten your arms.

Repeat these instructions for 15 repetitions and 3 sets.
Pull-ups concentrate on various muscle groups that burn more calories since several muscles including the biceps, triceps, back, and core are functioning simultaneously. This exercise may help you to become in shape, enhancing your capacity to burn fat and raising your metabolism. To accomplish a pull-up it practically needs 15 muscles and the key muscles are your lats and biceps.

According to the research, completing a pull-up routine can help you burn roughly 10 calories each minute. It is advised that at least 150 minutes of moderate-intensity or 75 minutes of vigorous-intensity activity ought to be done each week since cardio is one of the finest strategies to burn calories.

*Exercise Pattern*

Grip the pull-up bar with your arms completely extended by standing straight.
Now bend your knees and lift yourself till your chin clears the bar.
Come back to your initial posture carefully.
Repeat these instructions for 15 repetitions and 4 sets.

### *5. Squats*

Squat workouts are considered muscle-building exercises. The major purpose of this workout is to enhance the lower region of the body. Squats assist to burn calories and prevent fat from building in the lower area of the body. This workout helps enhance your mobility and also balance. A novice should strive for 3 sets of 12-15 repetitions of at least one form of squat to anticipate better results.

Exercise Pattern:

Stand straight with your feet wider than your hip width with your toes pointing front.
By bending your knees and ankles press your hips back.
Sit into a squat posture by keeping your heels and toes on the ground.
Keep your knees bent to a 90-degree angle and posture yourself parallel to the floor.
Straighten your legs by pushing your heels and return to the upright posture.

### *6. Lunges*

A popular strength training program that builds and tones your lower body and enhances overall fitness and sports performance. Lunges generally concentrate on strengthening your back, hips, and legs.

Lunges aid in strengthening lean muscle and reducing body fat. It is crucial to challenge yourself and use lunges in a high-intensity training regimen with the support of heavyweights. The single-leg motions featured in this exercise stabilize muscles to enhance balance, stability, and coordination.

*Exercise Pattern*

Stand straight with your back and abs upright.
Bend your knee by keeping your right leg in the front.
Now, bend your knee till your right thigh is parallel to the ground and your left one perpendicular.
Keep your front knee over your heel.

Come back and bring your feet together.
Repeat the same instructions with your left leg.
30 repetitions of alternating lunges are useful.
Along with activities that need to be done at your location for weight reduction. Some additional elements and strategies might be useful for weight control.

### *7. Yoga*

A 5000-year-old discipline has demonstrated to be a great weight reduction treatment. It is claimed to be invented by Rishis and Brahmans and contains 5 main principles: Exercise, Diet, Breathing, Relaxation, and Meditation.

The combination of Yoga and healthy eating has proved advantageous as it helps you shed weight along with keeping your body and mind healthy. It also enhances your consciousness and interaction with your body. You may also reduce your blood sugar levels by doing yoga for diabetes.

Along with weight reduction as a benefit, Yoga has other benefits to give such as:

- Improved Cardio Health
- Increased Muscle tone
- Balanced Metabolism
- Improved Respiration
- Increased Flexibility
- Stress Management

Yoga Poses are a vital aspect of weight loss. Yoga positions concentrate largely on boosting attention and developing your muscular tone. Your body should grow habituated to certain stances to generate optimum advantages from yoga.

Some of the yoga positions that should be done for weight reduction are:

- Warrior Pose
- Triangle Pose
- Shoulder Pose
- Bridge Pose
- Bow Pose
- Plank Pose
- Downward Dog Pose
- Sun Salutation

**Best time to workout**

Perhaps the greatest time to complete your regular exercise program is early in the morning. The fundamental reason for this is that exercising on an empty stomach is the greatest approach to burning stored fat.

Even though you feel upset by the early alarm clocks at first, it will progressively develop a habit for you, a healthy one at that. Say, you wake up every day at 7 am. This means your biological clock moves early, therefore making you sleepy quicker in the evening or at night. This assists in keeping the timetable rigorously.

However, there has been research that shows that doing out in the evening might be beneficial since our bodies consume lower oxygen during that time, which may assist boost our performance and in turn lose weight. Nonetheless, the studies are pretty restricted and the bulk of experts indicate morning is the favorite time to exercise if you wish to lose weight at home.

Follow these guidelines to make sure your weight-reduction plan at home is done properly:

Do not fall victim to fad diets that promise results in a short time.
Beware of appealing weight reduction pills and belts which may only deliver short-term benefits.
Starving oneself is not the appropriate option since it might lead to additional issues like acidity, sickness, etc.

# Chapter 6

## How to eat what you want and still lose weight

When it comes to achieving and maintaining a healthy weight, you might think you have to give up eating what you love. But that isn't the case. It's possible to eat your favorite foods and still achieve your weight-loss goals.

Here is a quick guide on eating in moderation and satisfying your cravings.

### *Portion control*

Perhaps the most important step of all in being able to eat what you love comes down to portion control. This might take some getting used to, but it can be an eye-opening experience to discover what an appropriate portion size really is.

And once you start practicing portion control and begin eating the right foods—in the right amounts—you'll soon find that a small serving of your favorite treat is all you need. You'll also learn tricks throughout the program that will help prevent you from overeating. For example:

Try to avoid eating foods straight from the package—which makes munching on multiple servings all too easy.

Instead, dish up a single serving and then place the package out of sight.

### *Savor the flavor*

When you eat your favorite foods, instead of devouring them in mindless gulps, try to slow down and allow yourself to really enjoy the moment, savoring each and every bite.

A fun way to practice mindful eating is with a piece of chocolate:

Sit down and take one small bite at a time.
Keep each bite in your mouth for a few moments before swallowing.
Notice the rich flavor, creamy texture, and intense sweetness.
You may be surprised at how one small piece of chocolate can satisfy a sugar craving when savored slowly.

### *Add movement and exercise to your day*

Exercise comes with many health benefits that range from relieving stress and improving memory to helping you sleep better. But when it comes to weight management, the real bonus is the speeding up of your calorie burn.

Knowing that you're burning a few extra calories allows you to enjoy a favorite food every now and then when you're craving it.

Whatever physical activity you choose, do it consistently. In addition to helping with weight loss, exercise can help improve happiness and also create the right mindset for eating healthier. There are plenty of great exercises you can do right from your home.

## Fill up on fruits and vegetables first

Fruits and veggies can be great compliments to the foods you love. Not only are they low in calories but they keep you feeling full and satisfied. So, when it comes to balancing your nutrition, always try to fill up on nutritious foods by starting with vegetables and fruits. Rather than eating your favorite candy on an empty stomach, eat a healthy meal first and save the candy for dessert.

You're likely to eat less candy. And, by saving the sugar for after your meal, you'll help to prevent your blood sugar levels from spiking. Adding fruits and vegetables to your diet is a lasting, meaningful habit that will help you live the healthiest version of your life.

### ***Cook the healthier version of what you love***

Sometimes, your favorite comfort foods just need a small tweak here and there to become healthier—but just as tasty—versions of themselves.

For instance, you could consider adjusting how you cook certain ingredients: Instead of deep-frying foods, try air-frying them! Another great way to upgrade what you're craving is by swapping for healthier ingredients: Try turning to fruit as a source of sweetness in baking rather than sugar. All you need is an open mind and a willingness to experiment in the kitchen.

**The bottom line:**

It's possible to continue to eat the foods you love and lose weight; it just comes down to balance. The saying, "Everything in moderation," may seem boring, but it's sage advice that works! Being able to have your cake and eat it— slowly, mindfully and in small amounts—allows you to develop a healthier long-term relationship with food.

Choosing to follow deprivation diets and avoiding all your favorite foods will only lead to weight regain when you can no longer resist the cake.

# Chapter 7

## Mental strategies to help lose weight

Motivation to reduce weight frequently reaches an all-time high when the first buds of spring break up, signifying that bathing suit season is not long behind. And although there's no getting past the need to exercise and eat properly, long-term weight reduction begins in your thinking. Experts suggest that having the appropriate mentality might help you imagine yourself as skinny.

If you want to succeed at weight reduction, you need to "reduce the mental fat, and that will lead to reducing the waistline fat," says Pamela Peeke, MD, author of Fit to Live. "Look at the patterns and behaviors in your life that you are carrying about with you that get in the way of achievement."

Everyone has their justifications. When attempting to change their lifestyle and nutrition, most individuals do OK until something occurs — whether it's job pressure, family troubles, or something else. Whatever your particular difficulty, the pattern has to alter if you want to be successful.

"I want to enable individuals to recognize these patterns, deal with the true causes, so they can go on and be able to succeed at healing their health," adds Peeke.

### *To Think Yourself Thin, Have Patience*

One key mental impediment to weight reduction is desiring too much, too soon. Blame it on our quick-gratification culture, with its instant texting, PDAs, and digital cameras: Weight reduction is too gradual to please most dieters.

"Losers seek instant results. ... Even though it took them years to acquire weight, once they start to lose weight, they have little patience with the suggested 1-2 pounds each week," says Cynthia Sass, MS, RD, a representative for the American Dietetic Association.

But you'll receive the finest outcomes when you lose weight slowly. Sass tells her customers that when they lose weight too rapidly, they're frequently shedding mainly water or lean tissue, not fat.

"When you lose lean tissue, metabolism slows down, making it much tougher to lose weight," she says.

### *Think Thin: 8 Strategies*

Get that overweight attitude out of your brain and start thinking like a skinny person with these eight strategies:

*1. Picture Yourself Thin.*

If you want to be skinny, envision yourself thin. Visualize your future self, six months to a year down the line, and think about how amazing you'll look and feel without the excess pounds. Dig out old images of your slimmer self and put them in a spot as a reminder of what you are aiming for.

Ask yourself what you did back then that you could put into your lifestyle now. And, suggests Peeke, think about things you would want to undertake but can’t due to your weight.

"To overcome old patterns, you need to perceive oneself favorably," Peeke explains.

*2. Have Realistic Expectations.*

When physicians ask their patients how much they want to weigh, the amount is frequently reasonably feasible. Peeke has her patients pick a realistic weight range, not a single figure.

"I ask them to think forward 12 months, and would they be happy being 12 or 24 pounds thinner?" she adds "It just amounts to 1-2 pounds each month, which is achievable, sustainable, and reasonable in the context of job and family." She proposes reevaluating your weight goal after six months.

*3. Set Small Goals.*

Make a list of minor objectives that will help you attain your weight reduction goals.

These mini-goals should be something that will enhance your lifestyle without wrecking devastation in your life, such as:

Eating more fruits and veggies every day.
Getting some type of physical exercise for at least 30 minutes a day.
Drinking booze solely on the weekends.
Eating low-fat popcorn instead of chips,
Ordering a side salad instead of french fries.
Being able to go up a flight of stairs without gasping for breath.
"We all know that change is hard and it is tougher if you attempt to make too many changes, so start small and gradually create lifestyle adjustments," recommends Sass.

*4. Get Support.*

We all need help, particularly during terrible times. Find a friend, family member, or support group you can connect with regularly. Studies reveal individuals who are connected with others, whether it's in person or online, fare better than dieters who attempt to do it alone.

*5. Create a Detailed Action Plan.*
Sass proposes that each night, you plan your nutritious meals and workout for the following day. Planning is 80% of the fight. If you're prepared with a comprehensive strategy, success will follow.

"Schedule your workout as you would an appointment," Sass adds. "Pack some dried fruits, vegetables, or meal replacement snacks so you won't be tempted to consume the incorrect sorts of things."

Make your health a priority by implementing such actions into your daily life, and eventually, these healthy activities will become a normal part of your existence.

*6. Reward Yourself.*

Pat yourself on the back with a trip to the movies, a manicure, or anything that will help you feel good about your successes (other than food rewards) (other than food rewards).

"Reward yourself once you have reached one of your mini-goals or dropped 5 pounds or a few inches around your waist, so you acknowledge your hard work and appreciate the measures you are doing to be healthy," Peeke adds.

*7. Ditch Old Habits.*

Old habits die hard, but you can't continue to do things the way you used to if you want to succeed at weight reduction.

"Slowly but surely, attempt to recognize where you are participating in habits that contribute to weight gain and turn them around with modest steps that you can easily do without feeling deprived," advises Sass.

For example, if you are an evening couch potato, start by changing your snack from a bag of cookies or chips to a piece of fruit. The following night, try having only a calorie-free drink. Eventually, you can start completing activities while you watch television.

Another method to get started abandoning your poor habits: Get rid of the tempting, empty-calorie meals in your kitchen and replace them with healthier ones.

*8. Keep Track.*

Weigh in often and maintain notebooks describing what you eat, how much you exercise, your emotions, and your weight and measurements. Studies demonstrate that keeping track of this information helps encourage beneficial habits and diminish negative ones. Simply knowing that you're monitoring your food consumption might help you avoid that slice of cake!

"Journals are a sort of accountability ... that assist to indicate which techniques are succeeding" explains Peeke. "When you are responsible, you are less likely to suffer food dissociations, or be 'asleep at the meal.'"

# Chapter 8

## How to overcome setbacks in weight losing

When on a weight-loss journey, setbacks are sure to occur. When they do, it is crucial to get back on track as fast as possible. This doesn't mean merely going on a diet, since diets are often supposed to be short-term. The idea is to concentrate on building a healthy lifestyle and way of eating that is not only possible but sustainable for the long term.

Changing one's lifestyle is not simple, and it doesn't happen immediately. It is an acquired skill set, and like most things in life it needs hard practice and the correct frame of mind. But once you commit to a lifestyle change and identify your objectives, you may take the initial steps.

### *Focus on what you are wanting to eat more of, not what you are trying to eat less of*

Instead of concentrating on eating less refined or processed meals and drinks, spend your time focused on adding more of the nutritious foods and beverages that you enjoy into your routine. It's considerably more probable that you will continue this over time as you'll love what you are eating rather than feel like you are missing out on something.

### *Change your atmosphere.*

Over time we all create routines. The longer we've been in a routine, the more difficult it is to change. The same is true with altering our dietary habits, to the point that we frequently don't know where to start. To start things moving, take a look at your surroundings and how you might make it simple to pick nutritious meals.

For example, if you are in the habit of dropping by a fast food restaurant every morning for breakfast and want to alter that practice, consider filling your fridge and pantry with healthy grab-and-go choices like hard-boiled eggs, Greek yogurt, cottage cheese, overnight oats, and protein drinks.

This simple adjustment of surroundings makes it easy to start the morning with a food victory.

***Incorporate physical activity that you enjoy into your day.***

Most of us feel better when we incorporate physical activity into our day, but oftentimes that physical activity can feel like a chore or, at times, even a punishment. Tailoring physical activity to what you enjoy can help you adhere to a more physically active lifestyle.

I enjoy dumbbell weights, resistance bands, and bodyweight movements for my strength training, while I enjoy walking and using a rowing machine for my cardio. Find what works for you and you'll find yourself looking forward to physical exercise rather than avoiding it.

***Take the time to plan and prepare.***

While many diets are short-term and not easily sustainable, there are options today that are less “diet” and more of a lifestyle change.

Mediterranean, ketogenic, paleo, vegan, low-fat, and low-carb are some examples. Often what makes these “diets" appealing and sustainable for the long term is the concept of meal planning.

One of the main predictors of success for someone looking to create a healthy long-term lifestyle is the mindfulness that is cultivated through the planning and/or prepping of meals.

This can be done through a combination of preparing food ahead of time for meals that will be consumed over the coming few days and incorporating some good quality pre-made meals from delivery services that fit your personal preference and lifestyle.

***Incorporate action-based forms of self-care into your routine.***

Most of us have many stressors in our lives and having tools to help dissipate the emotional tensions of our days is essential. So much of life is built on consumption-based activities — browsing the internet, our daily cup of coffee, perusing our social media feeds, watching television, smoking, drinking alcohol, snacking, and the list goes on.

As with most things in life, they should be done in moderation and balanced with action-based pursuits. Going for a stroll, volunteering or other acts of service, video chatting with a friend or family member, reading, having a massage, meditation, and starting up a new hobby are all examples of action-based activities that may help you decompress after a stressful day.

"Thanks for reading! If you loved this book or found it helpful I'd be extremely happy if you'd submit a brief review on Amazon. Your support truly does make a difference and I read all the reviews personally so I can gather your opinion and make this book even better.

Thanks again for your support!"

www.ingramcontent.com/pod-product-compliance
Lightning Source LLC
LaVergne TN
LVHW050316160826
845677LV00014B/3421

*9798359321655*